Perhaps You Do Not Know Who I Am

(Perhaps Neither Did I)

Rebecca Kopp-Dipiazza

Rebecca Kopp-DiPiazza

Perhaps You Do Not Know Who I Am
Perhaps Neither Did I

For information address:
Helm Publishing
3923 Seward Ave.
Rockford, IL 61108
815-398-4660
www.publishersdrive.com
ISBN 978-0-9801780-8-1

Printed in the United States of America

Dedication

In loving memory of my parents, Thelma Inez and Julius Christian Kopp, for giving me the greatest values in the world, integrity, faith, perseverance and compassion.

Acknowledgements

To my loving husband, Paul, who put his life on hold for the entire year. He literally allowed me to lean on him at every doctor appointment. He never complained of doing all of the errands and household chores.

To my three wonderful caring children Angela (who is an excellent compassionate nurse), Laurinda (Human Service Professional and who surprised me with the forward to this book) and Matthew (who is truly his namesake, a gift from God. He is the most caring and sensitive young man I have ever known.) They have supported me with their unconditional love and concern.

To my grandchildren Brian, Aeriel, Ashley, Kaitlyn, Nathaniel, and great-grandchild Zackery for bringing so much joy in my life.

To all of my brothers and sisters, Julius, Carolyn, John, Sandy, Judy, Sharon, Bob, Jeff and Greg, for believing in me when I doubted myself.

To my dearest friends, Shelley, Cheryl, and Colleen, for their many phone calls, visits and words of encouragement.

To Dr. Wolff and Maurtrice Williams MSW, for giving freely of their time to read the first manuscript.

My primary doctor, who never doubted me, and to Jennifer, my physical therapist who knew about my illness. She was truly an angel and educated me about my conditions and how I could help myself.

To Helm Publishing company and associates for their commitment and time to take my message and make it presentable to the public, especially Dianne Helm, my editor and publisher, who worked diligently with me to create this book.

I love you all. I am grateful to have you all in my life.

Perhaps You Don't Know My Mother

My mother is Rebecca Kopp-Dipiazza. She is a very strong and spiritual woman whom I admire. She taught me to be strong, have belief in myself and trust in the power of the Lord. Her strength stems from her spiritual background. Her faith has brought my entire family through some of the toughest valleys of our lives. This most recent valley that she has had to walk through has been the toughest for her. Let me help you understand why she made it through.

She has always gone to the Lord for her strength. She spends hours writing journals that speak of her trials and tribulations. Her journals are addressed to Dear Lord. Once I had the opportunity to listen to a few of her entries. She was very sad and worried for one of her children. Her concern and worry was evident in her writing. Reading the entry would have brought anyone to tears. That is how she would give her concerns to the Lord. She said that my grandpa always told her to speak to the Lord before she made any decisions and tell Him of her worries so that he could take them for her. He told her that by morning things would be clearer. That is exactly what she did, only instead of a simple prayer each time, she would journal instead. The amazing thing, is that the next day ,when she wrote in it again, her sorrow had fallen away and the only thing left was words that didn't even sound like hers anymore. I believe they were answers and directions from the Lord, with passages of hope and positive direction to guide her through whatever valley she was passing through at that time. The two entries of each sorrow were like night and day. One seemed to be written by her and the other by the spirit of the Lord. I have never been more amazed by the works of the spirit in her life.

She taught me to go to the Lord when I was down and He will help me through. She spent many days talking me through some rough times in my life. She listened to me late into the evening, talking and soothing, giving me insightful words of encouragement that could only have come from her years of wisdom gained from her spiritual guidance through life. She has taken a great amount of time from her life to listen to others wiser than her, to search out answers to her many questions, and to soak up as much knowledge that could help her become a better person. During her quest to become a better person, I have benefitted. She has shared many enlightening passages of wisdom that has helped me to become stronger and wiser too. Her mission in life is to educate others so that they may have more fulfilling lives and people may live together more peacefully. All she wants to do is to help others in any way that she can.

She has changed tremendously through her life and each change that she has made, has made her into a better person. For many years all she did was overextend her self in helping others. She would read, attend seminars, go to school, and work diligently. She wanted to be happy but more than that she wanted everyone else to be happy too. Over the years she has finally learned that she has to set boundaries in her life in order to survive. She has taught me about boundaries too. Although I am much like her and I struggle with those boundaries, I believe that I will be better at it because of her. She has taught me not to judge, to accept my children for who they are, love them and let them learn on their own. She has taught me to accept that not everyone will see things the way I do and there is nothing wrong with that. She has also reminded me that not everyone is on the same spiritual path and that is ok too. Most of all she taught me to forgive, not just because it is the right thing to do but because it is the best thing for my spirit. Inner peace only comes with forgiveness and faith. Many people will hurt us throughout our lives but only we can stop the pain. When we hold on to pain, it only hurts us more. She reminds me that anger is usually pain turned inward. Good things can come from terrible situations we just need to look for the good within the bad. My mom has found the good in every situation that she has encountered. In some instances it has taken her some time to find it but she always does. She has helped me to be a positive person.

She has always been a very giving person. I know that her spirit would not have had it any other way. She is a helper. She cares deeply for other people. She would give someone her own clothes if they would fit. She actually gave me hers once. She gave me some of her beautiful dresses so that I could be dressed professionally for business. That was back when I was first starting out and I was actually her size. She has been there to help all of our family members even to the extent of putting aside her own needs for herself. She gave money that she did not have, gave time that she needed for herself, gave up personal wants to give personal wants to others. Sometimes just to see someone smile she would get them something even if they didn't need it. She has always been about putting others first.

She is also the kind of person that can be depended on. She never goes back on her word. She is always there when you need her. Even when she was working she would not take a day off because she was concerned that her boss would not find someone to take care of the people that she took care of. She even went to work sick. She never took a day for herself unless she was sure that there was someone that was perfectly capable of handling whatever duty that she was responsible for at that time. The funny thing is that she always told me not to go into work when I was ill. She told me to always take care of myself first because if I didn't I would not be of any use to anyone. The only problem was that she never put herself first. There were many times that her friends and family would advise her to stop and take care of her own needs or her own health but she refused if it would cost anyone including her job any type of inconvenience. I don't think she ever felt that she was entitled to be first.

As a result of her unselfishness she has rundown her own physical body. You would think that this would destroy a person who was always moving, always helping, and always working. It did not destroy my mom. It tried. This event in her life was horrible but my mom made it through. She cried, worried, wrote, talked, and read. This could have broken her spirit and it nearly did. That is the key though, nearly. The Lord helped her through. He worked through all of those people who she held so dear to bring her strength, encouragement, love, concern, and even education. Even after she was betrayed by many, my mother still had the strength to forgive and still had the strength to abstain from passing judgment. She took responsibility for her own misfortune and learned from it. Now she has strong boundaries because the Lord put them there. She also has an opportunity to help others who might be going through the same things that she has gone through. She has also found the good inside of the bad just like always.

Laurinda Wittenhagen

Introduction

Through a veil of tears, I said to a physician, "Perhaps you do not know who I am." Thus, the title of this book was born. Within a twenty-four hour period from the onset of abdominal pain, urgency, and frequency to urinate, I became physically incapacitated.

I share my journey from the onset of the symptoms as I search for a medical diagnosis. The search took ten months, and visits with eight doctors to arrive at several diagnoses. The diagnoses are Interstitial Cystitis, Pelvic Floor Dysfunction, Irritable Bowel Syndrome, Bulging Disc, and Depression.

Each day I lived in fear and apprehension. My illness was invisible, my symptoms were invisible, and I felt invisible. My pain and deterioration were not validated. I was challenged mentally as I began to doubt myself. Deep inside, I knew that there must be a great gift in this challenge. I have always believed that within every adversity there is indeed a spiritual gift. Indeed, I found more than one gift.

It is my hope that sharing my story will give hope and inspiration to others who are facing a drastic life style change or illness. I believe my story would be helpful to medical and mental professionals as well.

Table of Contents

Interrupted

"What lies behind us and what lies before us are small matters compared to what lies within us."
Ralph Waldo Emerson

It was a normal Wednesday workday at the clinic. I must preset the medications for seventy clients. I must pull the charts of those who the doctor would see today. I had to insert the latest labs and make sure the doctor had room to write progress notes as well as orders. These of course are the normal duties of Wednesday. Having worked here for ten years, I could do all of these in a short amount of time. Today I do not feel well.

I am having pain in the lower abdomen. I palpate my bladder and it is tender and slightly distended. I have the urge to urinate. The employees' restroom is at the other end of the building. It seems the faster I try to walk, the more severe the pain. I slow down. This is difficult for me because my normal pace is a slow run. I finally make it. I try to empty my bladder but there is not much there.

Okay, I say to myself. This seems familiar to me. I will call my doctor and get an afternoon appointment. By that time the clinic doctor will be done, medications will have been administered and then I will see my doctor.

I complete my work slowly due to the pain, urgency and frequency to urinate. I realize I do not have the time to walk to the other side of the building; so, I use the client's restroom next door. I also call the part-time nurse, who works as a counselor, but would help me out should I need to leave sooner. I called my doctor and made an appointment for later in the afternoon.

I am sure the doctor will see me, check my urine, find no bacteria but will go ahead, as my previous doctors had, and prescribe me an antibiotic. I would be on my merry way back to work to finish the day. No such luck.

This doctor said, "You do not have a bladder infection." She palpates the lower abdomen, where the bladder is located, and I stifle a scream. She decides to do a pelvic exam. She states, "You have a cystocele. I will make arrangements for you to see an urogynecologist, and due to the chronic constipation I will also make an appointment for you to see the gastroenterologist. I cannot prescribe any pain medication. Try some ibuprofen." While I was there, she gave me a couple of pills. I had some ibuprofen at work. By the time I returned to work, the medication helped the pain.

The counselor/nurse came by to see how I was doing. I gave her the information. I said, "If I can make it through tomorrow. I will have Friday, Saturday and Sunday off to rest. Surely by that time, I will feel much better."

She said, "Remember, I have a conference to attend this weekend. You were supposed to take tomorrow off and work the weekend."

"Oh," I said, "well, that is better yet. If I can rest tomorrow, it should not be a problem." She left and I began to finish out the day.

I had to note the doctor's orders, change medication dosages, write progress notes, file the charts, balance the books, (which are the number of milligrams I dispensed for the day subtracting from the inventory), and secure the safe and the alarm for my office. This should have been completed in an hour and a half, but not today. I find I have to lay down several times with my feet and legs elevated. This seemed to give me some relief. I look at the clock and it is 7:00pm. I have been here over twelve hours.

As soon as I arrived at home, I told my husband I am not hungry and I just need to take a warm bath and relax. Afterwards, I told him about the day. He was concerned and understood that I needed to elevate my legs and go to bed. I thought after a good night's sleep, I would feel much better.

No such luck. I am up several times during the night to urinate. The pain is only dulled by the ibuprofen and I know I cannot take that every hour. Morning is here and I am exhausted. I cannot stand up straight. I am holding my abdomen as if that would take the pain away. I call my doctor and tell her, "Please, can you get me in to see someone today?"

"No," she says.

I say, "I cannot walk, sit or stand. The pain is so severe in my abdomen."

She told me she would call me back. She did get an appointment for the GI (gastroenterologist) the following week and due to the severity, the urogynecologist agreed to see me also. She said, "Keep your legs and feet elevated and continue to take the ibuprofen."

I have to call my supervisor; hopefully, he will find a nurse to help me. I said, "Please call the nurse we have on the board. I will come in and set up the medication and I will come in at the end of the day and close." I also said, "If she can't come in, get a nurse from the nursing pool and I will do the same. I cannot be there half a day much less all day."

He said, "I cannot justify hiring a nurse from the pool without a note from your doctor."

I said, "No problem." I called my doctor back and my husband got the note for me to give to my supervisor the next day. I was surprised my supervisor did not call me back. Surely, he would have a pool nurse there, if not the board nurse.

I walk into the clinic, go right to his office, hand him the note and ask him, "Where is my help?"

He said, "The board nurse told me that if you were in that much pain, you could hand the medication to a counselor and observe the counselor administering the medication as you sit in a chair."

I could not believe my ears! He knew perfectly well, I told him I could not sit, stand and hardly walk. I go to the restroom and then to the break room.

Here he comes as usual; this is our daily routine. We would have a cup of coffee and talk about problems or solutions related to the clinic. He sits down, looks me right in my face and says, "Is this really that bad?"

My eyes filled with tears and I say, "You people really do not care about anyone, do you?" Of course, I knew the answer to that. I had just finished working the holidays with the flu. I knew that a nurse had to be trained for two weeks at the least to be capable of doing my job. He knew as well as any of the administration that I have never called in sick. Then again, I had tolerated this behavior many times when I was sick; so, perhaps I should be called, "STUPID OR BETTER YET, MARTYR". After all, there had been a year, two, possibly more, when I worked five and a half days a week, some of which were ten hours a day.

Actually, my schedule was ten hours a day for four days a week and four hours every other Saturday. A part-time nurse was not easy to find for every Friday and every other Saturday. Previously I had worked part-time for two years and covered for the full-time nurse for vacation, personal days and illness. Evidently, I am not the usual person. What is that saying of Dr. Phil's? 'YOU TEACH PEOPLE HOW TO TREAT YOU!' That rings loud and clear now, especially, when I need help. The day only gets better!

Here I go shuffling off to the restroom, holding my abdomen, slightly hunched over and the CEO approaches me and asks, "Could you step into the office?" I hobble in still holding my abdomen due to the intense pain. He closes the door. My supervisor is sitting at his desk and offers me a chair. I brace myself as I try to sit. He asks, "Just what is the problem anyway?"

"Well," I put it bluntly; "I have a cystocele which is a protrusion of the urinary bladder and a rectocele which is a protrusion of the rectum, my bowels do not work, and I have severe pain of which I notified him yesterday," nodding my head toward my supervisor. "I called in yesterday and requested help and he said I needed a note from my doctor. He (supervisor) has it. I should be home with my feet and legs up per doctor's order. For some reason, the board nurse and my supervisor decided that I could sit in a chair while I watched a counselor administer the medication. I am actually surprised they did not find a way that I could lay on the exam table and administer the medication!"

"Oh, oh," he says looking at the supervisor. "Have you tried everyone?"

"Of course," he tells the CEO.

I cannot leave it alone. I said, "A pool nurse would have been very helpful; now, I know that was not even considered. Evidently, he and the board nurse decided what I was capable of doing." I stand; As far as I was concerned, the meeting was over. How dare them to question me! I have never called in sick and they both knew it.

"Who is scheduled to work tomorrow?" the CEO asks, as I am hobbling to the door.

I respond, "I am and I will. Next week I will not be here until my doctor releases me." I continue my day with many rest periods. I lie on the floor and elevate my legs and feet. I use the restroom next door. Frankly, I did not want to see my supervisor or CEO. I knew the sight of either one would make me angry. I needed to save my strength to finish the day.

Saturday I came in very early. I allowed time to preset the medications, and time for me to go to my sister's house so I can lie down until dispensing hours. Within ten minutes after my arrival to medicate, the CEO stops by to see how I am doing. He says, "You look great,"

I thought to myself, WOW WEE. He had no idea what I had to do to pace myself this morning. I replied, "Thank you." He made a quick exit. I told myself that I had to be accountable for I had allowed this treatment for years. That phrase by Dr. Phil, "You teach people how to treat you", says it all. There was no one to blame but me.

After I dispensed the medication, I lay on the floor and elevated my legs on my chair. I cried and cried. I made a promise to myself that day and it is still in place today. I would listen to my body and no one or job would ever be the priority. I had so many questions whirling through my head. What is wrong with me? Can I be fixed? How long would I be off work? Why do I have so much pain? I had no idea that these simple questions would go on for ten months. The nightmare had just begun.

Nonentity

"Let us treat men and women well; treat them as if they were real- perhaps they are."
Ralph Waldo Emerson

The search had just begun. I saw three specialists in my area along with my medical doctor. One was a gastroenterologist (GI doctor) who would be concerned about my bowels and why I do not have the urge to have a bowel movement. The second was an urogynecologist who would be concerned about the prolapsed bladder and the third specialist would be an urologist for a second opinion concerned with the urinary bladder.

The first visit was to the gastroenterologist (GI doctor). I asked him right away if the problem was because I had a major surgery, which resulted in the loss of my uterus, fallopian tubes and ovaries. I was curious about adhesions (scar tissue) which could constrict the bowel. He stated he did not think so since the surgery was many years ago. I did tell him about the pain in the lower abdomen that was inhibiting me from walking, standing up straight and sitting for more than thirty or forty minutes at the maximum. Then I would have to lie down with my feet and legs elevated, take pain medication and do nothing else for the day. He listened very patiently. He stated that he was going to try different kinds of medication as well as fiber, and he would also schedule some tests.

The fiber, as well as the medications, caused my abdomen to distend even more. He finally resorted back to using a natural laxative, as I had been doing in the past. The motility test proved I had colonic inertia (lazy bowel). The CAT scan was negative, no masses or constrictions were found. The colonoscopy proved I had irritable bowel related to chronic constipation. I was certainly thankful. I could live with this as I had been for the past seven years.

The urogynecologist visits and diagnoses led me on an emotional roller coaster. During the first visit, he diagnosed me with cystocele (protrusion of the urinary bladder), rectocele (protrusion of the rectum) and enterocele (protrusion of the small intestines)

"WOW"' I said. "No wonder I am having so much pain. My entire insides were protruding into the vaginal canal."

"No," he states. "These protrusions are not large enough for surgery and are not responsible for the pain. I want to do another test. Make an appointment at the desk for Thursday."

My husband and I return on Thursday as scheduled. We had talked about what the doctor said at the first appointment. I asked my husband to come into the exam room with me. I was not confident enough due to the pain, that I could retain everything the doctor would say. The nurse led us to the exam room and then told my husband to wait in the lab area until the doctor completed the test. I reiterated to her that it was important that my husband is present to hear the results.

The doctor walks in, hands me a scorecard and says, "The pain scale is from one to four. One is the lowest pain and four is the highest. I will be instilling three different fluids and I want you to score each one when I ask."

The first fluid I gritted my teeth and said, "Three. The second fluid I forgot all about the score card and said, "Ten! Please take it out!"

He said, "The next fluid I instill is a medication that will help the irritation in the bladder. You must try to hold the medication in the bladder for twenty minutes to get the maximum affect of the medication."

He stood up and said, "You have a severe case of interstitial cystitis, which is an inflammation of the bladder lining." He proceeded talking as he washed his hands at the sink. He stated, "There are only two treatments available for this condition. One is that I will prescribe a pill that you will take three times a day. The second treatment is instilling a combination of medications directly into the bladder. I want to start this next week. Schedule two appointments weekly with me for the next four weeks. If you do not respond to the treatments, I will send you to physical therapy." Before I could say another word, he opens the door, the nurse shoves some pamphlets at me and she exists with the doctor.

I am shocked. They left and did not talk with my husband. What did he say I should do? Oh, I remember, something about holding the medication in my bladder for twenty minutes and to schedule two appointments a week for four weeks. Both the doctor and nurse had simply discharged me.

I find my husband in the lab area waiting to see the doctor. He said, "What happened? Where is the doctor?"

I said, "I am totally confused. I will tell you in the car. I have to make appointments for the next month." He can tell by my voice that I am very irritated. I tried to talk to him in the car; but the bladder spasms were so severe, I could not explain anything. I asked him, "Will you please stop at my sister's house? I need to lie down. I cannot tolerate the ten mile drive to our house. I want to empty my bladder as soon as possible." We stopped at my sister's house. I emptied my bladder after the twenty minutes. I thought the cramping would stop. It did not. I knew I just needed to get home, lie down and elevate my feet and legs.

After we got home, I tried to read the pamphlets, but I could not concentrate. I took a couple of ibuprofen. I realize now that it has been two hours and the bladder is continuing to cramp. Now, I am angry. Why didn't someone tell me about this? I have never had bladder instillations. Surely, the medical professionals who work in this area should know this.

I make a call to the doctor's office. I tell the receptionist to have this particular doctor's nurse call me back not when she has one minute, but only when she can take her time. I also stated, "I do not deserve to have pamphlets shoved at me. I am sick and I am in pain. I want some answers!" The receptionist assured me that the nurse would get the message.

When the nurse returns the call within an hour I ask, "Why wasn't I informed about this continued cramping?"

"Everyone responds differently," she says and then proceeds to answer the questions I have about the procedure. She also said, "The answers to the questions you have asked are in the pamphlets I gave you. Evidently, you did not read them."

DING! DONG! She does not get it! I said, "I do not think you understand. I was unable to focus on pamphlets because I am in PAIN."

Evidently she got the message. Her voice softened and said, "The doctor will call in a prescription for your pain."

Finally, I have been heard and only because I had demanded it. I also found out the doctor would see my husband and me when I made an appointment. She transferred me to the appointment desk. The doctor would be out of town and he was very busy for the next two weeks. By the time we could see the doctor it would be near my last bladder instillation.

I cooperated and kept my appointment for the bladder instillations. I asked the nurse, "Do any of your patients with IC (Interstitial Cystitis) have the same symptoms? Are they able to do normal activities?"

She responded, "Everyone is different."

This must be her standing answer to everyone. The doctor came in and I asked him, "Doctor why my energy level is so low?"

He stated, "I do not treat energy levels."

I could not believe what he just said. I wanted to scream. Am I the only one who suffers with the cramping? Am I the only one who is unable to do anything but exist? What is the big secret? I just lay there on the exam table, tears rolling down my cheeks while they make their quick exit. I feel hurt. I do not know what to think. I start to wonder if I am not crazy. I certainly am confused.

Are they treating me like this because I am a nurse and they must be careful about giving me any information? I have worked long enough in the medical profession to know that some nurses would say, "Be careful with this patient. There is a nurse in his/her family, say as little as possible and document well, dot every "I" and cross every "t".

In the meantime, I got busy on the computer for the short intervals my body would allow. I located the Interstitial Cystitis Association. I left personal information with them so they could contact me. I found information on prolapses. I knew one thing for sure, if I was going to learn anything about my conditions, I better do my own research.

The next day as I lay on the sofa, I feel guilty watching my husband do all of the chores. He is not well either. In fact, I had been doing the yard work and mowing. Now I could not sit on a mower. I could not sweep. I could not mop. Any type of movement would cause cramping in the bladder or in the abdominal muscles. Walking up or down stairs was out of the question. I am depressed and confused. Just everything was on my mind. I had no answers or solutions. When anyone called me from work, all I could say was that I am continuing to have pain. I am having bladder instillations and I am taking medication.

That night I received a call from a woman in Virginia. She was connected with the Interstitial Cystitis Association. She asked me how I was feeling. I had a lot to say. She was diagnosed several years ago with interstitial cystitis. When I told her about the pain, prolapses and constipation, she validated the feelings and stated she had degenerative disc disease, fatigue syndrome, irritable bowel, and interstitial cystitis.

After I told her my story and the frustrations, she said, "It sounds like your doctor is not acquainted with the symptoms that affect other parts of the body. Just give me a moment and I will check to see if there is a doctor in your area that belongs to the Interstitial Cystitis Association." She looked on a list of doctors that were in the Association. She could not find one in my area. She did say, "Your symptoms that you are having now are closely related to symptoms of pelvic floor dysfunction. Has your doctor arranged for physical therapy?" I said, "No, but he did mention something about physical therapy if I did not respond to the medication and to the bladder treatments."

She asked for my address to send me information about the symptoms of interstitial cystitis and how it affects other areas of your body. She also told me that most of the people she has met with interstitial cystitis and pelvic floor dysfunction have had a history of hysterectomy. She explained that the pain was probably in the pelvic floor muscles. She assured me that what I was experiencing was justified. I could not wait to receive the information.

I continued receiving the bladder instillations and I would not say a word. Finally, I received the information in the mail. I had to go for a bladder instillation. For the past three bladder instillations, I kept quiet. I did not ask any questions. Now I had the information, so I courageously ask the doctor, "Why am I not able to work?"

He states, "I don't know. I did not say you could not work. My other patients work." I persisted, "Why do I have this pain in my bladder, pelvis, or abdominal muscles?"

He responded, "I have no idea why or where you have pain. Maybe you have a hernia. I will drop your doctor a note." I could not believe what he just said. I sat up as soon as he instilled the medication and I said, *"Perhaps You Do Not Know Who I am.* I have worked all of my life and for the last twenty-six years as a nurse. I have raised a family. I have worked two jobs at times. I did not walk; I ran. I did not sit down to return patient calls I stood. Now since this illness has happened to me I cannot work. I cannot stand up straight, walk much faster than a snail, and whether you believe me or not I have pain!"

Again he reiterates, "I will drop your doctor a note." The doctor and nurse make their quick exit as usual.

I made an appointment with my medical doctor so she could check my progress which was very little if any. I also tell her that my lower back hurts. She orders a MRI of my lower back. I told her that the urogynecologist thought I might have a hernia. We knew the CAT scan was negative. I could tell by the look on her face that she was not impressed. She asked me if I would see one more specialist in town for a second opinion; I agree. She makes the appointment with a reputable urologist in town.

Before the appointment with the Urologist, I have completed my bladder instillations and have taken the medication long enough to know that I was not responding. The Urologist examines me and finds that the prolapses are "normal for a woman of my age." He did not have any idea why I was having pain. I told him about the interstitial cystitis. He groped for words to describe the treatment. I explained what had been done. He wished me good luck. He made it very clear that he did not treat interstitial cystitis.

Over two months had passed. I remained in the dark about my pain. I have been diagnosed with irritable bowel related to chronic constipation, colonic inertia (lazy bowel), prolapsed bladder, rectum, and small intestine and interstitial cystitis; not one of these specialists knew why I was having the pain or cramping that was inhibiting me from normal activities.

I know my job is not going to wait forever. I also know family medical leave is for three months. I have used the majority of sick time, personal time and vacation. I have no answers to when I can resume my normal life or if I ever will. As my husband said to me, "The doctors have not determined you are disabled."

Yes, my husband is right. Not one doctor has told me I am disabled. However, I do have an appointment with rehabilitation. I wonder how this is going to help me. This doctor must know more than he is telling me; otherwise, why would he send me to rehabilitation? Again he is not the type of doctor that likes questions. He evidently does not like to educate his patients. I wonder if rehabilitation is his last ditch effort of treatment. At this point, I do not care what he says. There are still many questions unanswered. Getting answers from this doctor was like a dog chasing his tail.

Now I decide I must find specialists, in other areas, even if that means going to another state. I have not been comfortable with this doctor from the very beginning. I needed to be reassured that I am receiving the proper treatment or if there is new treatment available. I had the phone numbers of the two clinics I would consider. Upon arriving home I called both clinics. So what if the appointments could be a month or more away, that is one thing I had was time. In the meantime, I had to go to rehabilitation just as the doctor ordered.

Validation

"The soul always knows what to do to heal itself. The challenge is to silence the mind."
Carolyn Myss

I had no idea how rehabilitation would help me. Of what, or how, would be news to me. I did know that rehabilitation or physical therapy would help those who have been injured or have had surgery. The urogynecologist is the doctor who ordered physical therapy and all I could recall from one of his vague answers was something about strengthening the muscles. I did not know if he was talking about the abdominal muscles or the pelvic muscles and how this would be accomplished. Well as you can probably guess by now, either the doctor did not know himself, or he was not a teacher and or did not have time to waste talking about details.

I am hopeful this will not be the case with the therapist for physical therapy.

I am fifteen minutes early for the appointment to fill out the necessary papers and insurance information. I heard my name being called just as I completed the paperwork. She introduced herself and shook my hand. I could already feel the warmth emanating from the large smile on her face.

I can't help but notice she is at least six months pregnant. It was like a light bulb had lit up. I bet she can understand the pain I have. If she has other children, she would know what labor pains were. My pain was similar to labor pains.

She led me to her office and said, "Describe the pain and rate it on a scale of one to ten." "Eight," I said. "Lying down and elevating my legs and feet, I maintain pain at two or three. It really depends on how long I have been up and what activities I have done. I have been on my feet for forty-five minutes before I got here. I have done nothing except walk in the store and get a couple of items before I came here." I watched her as she wrote in the file. She was very conscientious. I could tell she was very interested in my past history and especially of the vertical scar she observed on my abdomen.

The exam began with an electrode she introduced into the vagina and the electrode was connected to a computer. I did not ask questions; I did not have to. She explained the results of the test. She had me lie down and then stand up. The readings she obtained were of the pelvic floor muscles. She stated that the number the computer gave her should be the same when lying down as compared to when I was standing. Mine were abnormal.

The number standing was much higher than the one in the resting position. She explained that she needed to enter the vaginal canal to examine the pelvic floor muscles. When she touched any one of those muscles I almost jumped off the table. She apologized. I told her I would be okay and I could stand the pain so she could get all of the information she needed.

Afterwards, she said to me, "The muscles should be soft and supple. Yours are like guitar strings. They are like tight bands with knots on them." I want to yelp with joy. She had actually found THE PAIN. I am not crazy. I am not imagining it. "Thank you! Thank you! You have no idea what this means to me. I have been to several doctors and they continued to tell me their other patients did not complain of pain and if I did have pain they did not know where it was or why."

With a puzzled look on her face, she said, "I want to massage the muscles two times a week. This will be painful. You need to take your pain medication thirty minutes before the visit."

I asked, "Have you seen other people with my condition?"

"Yes," she answered.

So I asked, "Did your other patients have histories of hysterectomies or abdominal surgery?"

Again she said, "Yes, some have had hysterectomies and some had interstitial cystitis. So if at any time you need to use the restroom, it will not be a problem."

I was so pleased to hear that she was knowledgeable about my condition. I asked her about her education and she informed me that she had special education to do this type of work. She stated there is one other therapist in this area and she worked out of a hospital. My gosh, I say to myself, she is truly an angel.

She validated my pain and understood about interstitial cystitis, what more could a person ask? She was open and answered questions and even referred me to some reading material that would help me to understand more of the physics of my condition. She told me the name of the book is *A Headache in the Pelvis*.

The first month of therapy I continued to walk in a stooped position holding my abdomen. I did not care that I hurt after the session. I was confident she knew what she needed to do, and I believed in her.

I am not saying that psychologically I was totally wonderful. Sometimes, I would lie in the darkness of her office with the heat packs on my abdomen after a session and cry. I cried for my life as it was before this illness. I cried because I did not know if I would ever go back to that life. No one knew the answers to that question, not even the therapist. I had to walk one step at a time like a blind person groping in the dark for something to hold on to.

I will tell you that after ten weeks of therapy and learning about relaxation methods by using biofeedback that I could relax the muscles for short periods of time. I used the deep breathing also to help empty the bladder completely. I could stand up straight and walk; although, the maximum time on my feet, whether standing or walking, was limited to forty-five minutes. I was grateful for this therapist. She recognized when my progress had ended; although, I had an open invitation to come back should I feel the need.

Around five weeks into the physical therapy, I got a disturbing call from work and many disturbing calls from the short-term disability insurance offered through my job.

Interrogation

"There must always remain something that is antagonistic to good."
Plato

Human resources called to ask if I had received any checks from the short-term disability insurance. "No", I said. "A lady called me about two weeks ago and stated she would be the person who would be handling my claim."

Human resources stated, "You should have received a couple of checks by now. I will call them to make sure they have everything they need. I have called to let you know that your family leave of three months has expired. The administration has decided to give you an extra month. So, at the end of this month, we need a note from your doctor telling us if you can return or not. We can no longer hold your position after that."

I said, "I understand completely. I am so thankful that you have been so patient with me for as long as you have. I am still in the dark myself. I have been going to rehabilitation. I have also made appointments with other specialists out of the area; but they will not be for a couple more months. Be assured by the end of this month, I will have the doctor say one way or the other if I am capable of returning to work."

The lady from the insurance company calls and gives me her name, telephone number and extension. She states that the reason the insurance company has not sent me any money is because they cannot determine if I am disabled. She is looking at my medical doctor's records and asked why I canceled an appointment. "What are you talking about?" I asked. She gives me the date and I get my calendar. Right away I know what she means. I inform her that I did not cancel. I had made the appointment to ask a question. My doctor's nurse called back and gave me the answer. The nurse also told me that the appointment would not be necessary. I gave her information to obtain records from the other doctors I have seen, as well as my visits to physical therapy.

Again, a week goes by and I hear nothing from the insurance company. So I call them and she said, "The urogynecologist has not sent your records."

I tell her, "No problem. I will call medical records." Tracy is in charge of medical records.

This would be the first of four calls from me that she would get. In fact, we became so acquainted that she said to me, "You have worked hard all of your life. What is the problem with the insurance company? You deserve disability and they are just dragging their feet." How correct she was.

Tracy had faxed my records twice and had mailed them with next day delivery. The insurance company said, "Perhaps the records got lost in the mail." They stated the fax was in another building. The last time, Tracy called the insurance company and told my insurance representative to stand by the fax machine. Tracy also told them she would not fax or mail any more records without a fee. The long lost records had been found and another two weeks had passed.

Now, I had to wait for their medical clientele to decide whether I am disabled or not. Whatever they decided would determine if I qualified for short-term disability.

In the meantime, I received many more calls questioning me about my condition such as, "Why did you refuse surgery?"

I say again, "What are you talking about? I was told by two different specialists that I am not a candidate for surgery."

"Well, our medical staff thinks that if you had surgery you could go back to work," she states. I want to scream out loud.

I have had enough of this nonsense, I say, "Look lady, I have three prolapses that are not operable. I have a bowel that does not work on its own. I have interstitial cystitis and the muscles in the floor of my pelvis do not do their job either. I am sick. I am in severe pain and I am tired of your interrogations. I suggest if you have any more questions, call my doctor. I am not interested in what you or your nurses think."

She must have got the message. I did not receive any more phone calls.

In fact, human resources called and asked if I received any money from the short-term disability. I told her everything I had been through. She said, "I wished you would have called me. I would have been glad to take care of that situation."

"I had no idea," I said, "I thought by cooperating, the insurance company would actually expedite the claim."

Needless to say, the insurance company did not care who I was or what I was going through. They did not respect me as a human being. They, like so many others, objectified me. If they could find that I was lying, I suppose they would have saved their company some money.

Human resources checked into the matter and called me right back. She said, "There will be a large check mailed within two days to you. You should have been paid eight weeks ago. If you do not receive it, call me within the week." I did receive a check in the mail. Now the decision had to be made by my doctor whether or not I was capable of working.

I was sitting in the exam room waiting for my doctor. Today is the day. A decision has to be made. I knew what the answer would be, but a part of me kept that at bay. The doctor enters the room and I tell her I need a note stating whether or not I can return to work. She and I know the answer, but the formalities must be followed. She handed me the note and walked out of the room. I started crying. Even though I knew this was the reality of my situation, I had been so busy seeking answers and defending myself, I had not had the time to think about grieving.

The realization that I no longer could anticipate going back to my job was like losing a family. I loved my job, the staff and the clients. I gave myself a little time to get myself together before I left the doctor's office.

I reminded myself that I have two other doctor appointments to attend and even though I could not return to my job, I could not give up, not now anyway.

Stuck

"All things come round to him who will but wait."
Henry Wadsworth Longfellow

I have not completed my physical therapy. Progress has been slow but beneficial. The appointment with one of the most reputable universities had arrived. The clinic was less than one hundred miles but it may have well been one thousand miles. The bumps in the road due to the road construction had no mercy on me. Even though I medicated myself before the drive, I was in severe pain by the time we arrived.

The receptionist gave me the necessary forms to fill out. I could not sit, my abdomen was so distended. I could not stand without the abdomen cramping. It was too early to take any medication. I hopped from one foot to the other while I leaned against a window ledge.

The doctor was punctual. The nurse leads my husband and me to the exam room and completes the usual duties. She weighs me, takes my temperature, blood pressure and leads me to the restroom to give a urine specimen. This was very much welcomed. I had to use the restroom on an average of ten to fifteen times a day.

The doctor enters the room. I tell her about the distention of the abdomen if I sit, stand or walk for more than forty minutes, and the cramping in the abdomen that radiates around to and including the lower back. She observed that I was in pain now. I told her about the interstitial cystitis. She is not interested and stated she was more concerned about the pain.

She said, "I want to give you some medication. I will inject the medication into your side muscle. This muscle is known as "the joker of pelvic pain", if your pain is alleviated by this, it will tell me that your pelvic pain is referred rather than in the pelvis."

Ample time had passed. She enters the room and she knows by the look on my face that the pain is not gone. She says, "Well at least I know it is in the pelvic floor muscles."

She examines me and hits the trigger points of the muscles. It was all I could do to stay on that table. I wanted to scream. She acknowledges that the pelvic floor muscles need physical therapy.

She suggests that I stay at a hotel for a couple of weeks in the city. She explains that she would inject medication into the pelvic muscles that would numb them enough so a therapist could massage them for a longer period of time. Otherwise, what I was getting from my therapist was okay but would take a longer period of time to stabilize the pain. She said if we decided to stay in the city to let her know and she would set up the appointments.

My husband and I talked about it on the way home and we agreed I would continue the therapy in our town rather than stay in the city. Time was not a factor to be considered. My therapist was seeing me twice a week and I medicated myself before each session. There was nothing to gain as far as I was concerned.

After another month had passed, it was time to go to the clinic in another state. I had progressed as far as possible with physical therapy. I continued to have pain upon any activity. At least I could stand up straight when I walked and have learned how to manage the pain with medication and relaxation techniques.

This particular clinic had many specialists. I had spoken to a nurse about who I should see. I gave her all of the information regarding my case. She would talk with the doctor and they would decide whom I should see. I was positive this appointment would be the one that would solve my problems, or at least tell me how to help myself.

No such luck. I was scheduled to see a regular gynecologist. He asked the same standard questions. He flipped through all of my medical records. He did a pelvic exam, then states, "Your problems are complex. You will have to come back and see at least three other doctors."

This was what I did not want to happen. That is why I spoke to a nurse to make the appointment. "Is there any way I could see these other doctors today?"

"I am not sure." He leads us to the appointment desk. There are three receptionists at this desk. The doctor tells one of them who he wants me to see. Immediately I was told that one of the doctors was not there and the other two are booked for two months. I stood there for ten minutes and finally say, "I have got to sit down."

She explains that it will take her awhile to find an appointment with the three doctors that would correlate. After another thirty minutes, she calls my name. I go up to the desk. She hands me two pages of appointments including lab tests. The appointments are scheduled two months away.

Perhaps You Do Not Know Who I Am

I cannot believe it. What in the world is it going to take for me to get it through my head that what is going on with me is not that simple? I am tired, in pain and very irritated. My husband was also, so we agreed, "what a wasted trip."

I realize by the time I come back for these appointments it will be ten months that I have been stuck. Yes, stuck in a rut going from doctor to doctor. It is time for me to wake up and smell the coffee.

I have got to learn to go with the flow. There is no magic pill or surgery.

Irritable and Isolated

"You cannot or will not encounter a circumstance or a single moment that does not serve directly and immediately of your soul to heal"
Gary Zukav

As I said earlier, I had two months before my last consultations. My time had been used running to doctor appointments and attending therapy for three months, of which I had reached a plateau. The therapist and I decided that should I need her at anytime all I needed to do was ask my doctor for the order. Now it was time to see how I could live around my pain.

I spent many hours crocheting, working jigsaw puzzles, reading and listening to music. I practiced relaxation methods and breathing deeply as the therapist had taught me. On some days I actually believed I was healed.

So I decided to get out of the house. Doing the activities I had been doing and going from the sofa to the recliner was okay for a time.

I began to feel like my world was shrinking and I was becoming more and more isolated. I thought, just maybe, if I could get out to the store or the bookstore, which I loved, I would feel much better, and who knows? Maybe I could strengthen those muscles and cure myself. After all, no one had told me any different. In fact, the doctors I spoke with told me, if anything, this would just take time. They did not say how much time or that I would have good days and bad days. I was not aware that at times I would believe I was healed.

My first excursion was to a large department store. I knew there were benches available. I knew where the restroom was. After all, I had to urinate from ten to fifteen times a day and if I tried to avoid the urge; the cramps would get severe. I took my pain medication before I left home. I walked slowly from the parking lot telling myself to take plenty of time. Do not be in a hurry. Just enjoy yourself.

I got inside the store and headed for the health and beauty section. I was not there ten minutes before I had to go to the restroom. The pain had started in the abdomen. After emptying my bladder, I was sure I was good for another thirty minutes so I walked to another department. Here we go again! I am irritated because now the pain is radiating around to the low back. I put whatever I had in my hands back and left. By the time I got home it was still too soon to take any medication. I got my pillows and welcomed the sofa. That's okay, I said to myself. I will go again another day, or next week.

The following week I decided to go to the bookstore. I loved bookstores and especially this one. It had sofas and big comfortable chairs to sit and read. Most of all, I had all the time in the world. This time I did not take any medication until I arrived. I found the restroom right away. Afterwards, I went to my favorite section of the store. I was interested in several books, so I took three to the big comfortable chair in the corner. I read for a while and chose the one I would buy. As I walk to the front of the store the pain in the abdomen began. I saw the long line of people and knew I had to get home. Again that sofa I detested began to look like a dear friend.

I did enjoy the outings even though they were short.

I also found I could visit my family and be comfortable. They were very aware of my condition and knew I would need to lie down and elevate my legs. It was encouraging because I had a wonderful visit and enjoyed being in different surroundings.

Psychologically I was not doing as well as I thought. I started waking up during the night crying. I would get up and think about what I had dreamed. Most of the time I dreamed I was homeless.

I was afraid I could not survive. I tried to appease myself with comments like, "You'll get better. It just takes time." How much better and how long will it be to return to my old self? Not one of the doctors could answer that question. I obsessed about other comments like, "Is it really that bad?" or "You look great", or "Just maybe she is pretending to be sick so she can take the vacation she had planned."

I read the progress notes of all of the doctors I had seen in this area. The urogynecologist was the one I was most upset about. He said in so many words that I took a lot of his time and his nurse's time asking questions regarding how long I would be disabled (to which he stated I was not). He insinuated my pain was questionable. He did not see any reason why I could not perform normal activities. Why am I surprised? The man did not believe me from the beginning; my instinct had told me that! He had also told me he was the only doctor in this area that treated interstitial cystitis.

The more I thought about the diagnosis of interstitial cystitis, I recalled working for an urologist. During my training, a middle-aged woman came in. I never got a chance to work with her because the office was so busy and I needed to be taught about biofeedback. Only the seasoned nurses could do biofeedback. I recall the comment made about her. The nurse told me this lady had interstitial cystitis.

She went on to say that this lady was a big "cry baby". She goes on to say, "she complains of every little pain even when her bladder is not full." Now it dawns on me why, when I mentioned interstitial cystitis, the doctors would evade discussing this particular diagnosis. I am not crazy. These doctors I have been seeing have formed their own definition and prejudices about this disease. Even the doctor who professes to be the only one in town who treats the disease is not convinced a person has pain and can become disabled.

I was getting angrier and angrier. I felt I was on a battlefield fighting for the right to be heard. One time I even snapped at my sister. I was tired of being asked, "How are you?" I told her, "Please do not ask me that anymore. I am in some form of pain at all times. I am so frustrated and irritable with myself and this illness."

I finally had to face what no one was telling me. I had several chronic problems. They were not going to heal. I would have to learn to live around the limitations or be prepared to deal with the consequences at this time. I still had hope that the appointments with the three doctors at the clinic would have a better answer. Maybe they had done further research on my conditions, or maybe they would educate me on some other things I could do to help myself.

The miracle appointment arrived. As before, my husband and I went a day earlier because of the distance. I saw an internal medicine doctor first. He took my history and discussed the findings of my previous doctors. He ordered some labs to be done and then I was to see the urologist. The urologist findings were the same. The prolapses were not bad enough for surgery and he evaded talking about the interstitial cystitis. The next appointment was with an urogynecologist and he was very busy. We waited three and half hours to see him. He saw me for fifteen minutes. He advised physical therapy. The next appointment was back to the same gynecologist I saw in September. I told him we are thirty minutes late to see the internist. He assured me to go on. He did not have any more to tell me from his exam in September.

The internist said, "Your labs are great. You are low in vitamin D. He gave me a prescription. He told me I did not have an autoimmune disease. He suggested that I stay in the city and receive physical therapy. I ask, "What is the difference where I go for physical therapy?" He said, "You would be injected with medication so that the therapist could be more aggressive in massaging the pelvic floor muscles." He went on to say that he was very well acquainted with "people like me" and went further to explain that I have overworked my body for a long time and now the body needs rest. He patted me and said, "You will get better in time. It took a long time for you to get to this point and it will take a long time for you to feel better." There we go again with that phrase, "you will get better in time" and yet, not telling me just when that is.

I think about what the lady from Virginia had said to me, "Sounds as if you may have pelvic floor dysfunction." She is absolutely right on. That is exactly what is I have. Surgery or medication does not cure this. My well being depends on how I listen to my body. This was a whole new area for me.

Belief System

"A man cannot be comfortable without his own approval."
Mark Twain

I waited for one week before I contacted my medical doctor. I did not want to see her until she had a report from the last clinic. She had all the records from all of the doctors. She said, "You have seen many doctors for a consult and now, it is time for you to get some rest. Should the pain get so bad and you need to go back to physical therapy, I will order it for you. Otherwise, I will continue to order your medication for you as you need it refilled."

She, of all doctors, knew me the best. She knew when I came to see her it was on my lunch hour from work. She also knew that I would work regardless of how I felt. She is right. I needed to rest. It has been ten months now and I had pursued ten doctors including her, and that did not include the rehabilitation therapy I attended for three months.

Actually, at six months I had progressed as far as I could. My income from sick pay, vacation pay and short-term disability was over. I applied for social security. I was denied in six weeks. I appealed and again I was denied within six weeks. Now, here I am at ten months and I know I need to hire an attorney.

I told my doctor about the denials and she encouraged me to do whatever I needed to do. She did, however, ask me what diagnoses I had given social security. I told her and finally, she, of all of these doctors, gave me the correct diagnoses. Not to say that I did not have interstitial cystitis, prolapses, irritable bowel related to constipation, slighted bulging disc, but that I also had pelvic floor dysfunction. What did she say?

Now, I remember where I heard that term, pelvic floor dysfunction, it was from the lady from The Association of Interstitial Cystitis.

I did my homework and found information on pelvic floor dysfunction. Interstitial cystitis and pelvic floor dysfunction have similar symptoms and often are diagnosed together. Pelvic floor dysfunction is when the muscles of the pelvis tighten and will not allow the bladder to empty and also affects the muscles of the rectum causing constipation. Actually even my bulging disc affects the nerves connected to the bladder. I read that muscle relaxants are given along with laxatives to relieve the constipation to avoid more pain from the pelvic muscles. I was taking muscle relaxants, laxatives and pain medication.

My next step was to pursue disability. I knew this was a lifelong disease.

I hired an attorney. I gave him all of my medical records and my two denials from social security. The attorney told me this could easily take up to one more year to get a court date. I told him a year compared to the rest of my life was not that long.

Now it was time for me to integrate my life with my illness. I knew it was time to accept my illness. This was easier said than done. I continued to wake up crying. If I wasn't crying, I was depressed. I decided I needed to leave myself alone and recognize that I was grieving and that all of these feelings were natural. Somehow I suppressed the anger.

My life as I knew it was gone. A great deal of my identity was gone; my body had physical limitations. My financial independence was gone and that, probably more than anything, affected my pride.

Oh how I wanted someone or something to blame! Referring to my job, a friend stated, "They did this to you." My sister felt the same way. She and my friend had seen me at work many times when I was sick. I wanted to delight in their anger and believe that this was justifiable. I had to tell them not to be angry. Intellectually, I knew the only one to blame was myself; emotionally, however, I did not believe that. I thought about all of the comments that were made about me and I obsessed about them.

"How dare those people to talk about me like that! I was a good, loyal employee."

I was also upset with the doctor who diagnosed me with interstitial cystitis. I had the opportunity to read his progress notes and he was very clear to say that there was no way that I should be incapacitated.

I remembered very well what my husband said, "The doctor has to say you are disabled and he has not said that." Yet, I was the one whose body had crashed. I also recalled my husband saying to me in the courting days, "The one thing that concerns me is that you do not care about yourself." I also had heard that from another man I had dated. That particular comment bothered me the most. Where did they get this message that I do not care about myself?

Other comments by my husband were, "You should not go to work sick. It is the company's business to replace you." Actually, before this happened I was trying to find a nurse to work for me for a vacation I was going to take in March. That was stressing me because I had already paid for the trip to Paris, France and my supervisor was not helping me to find someone I could train before it was time for me to go.

The job I had, although it required a nurse, did not require the general duties a nurse would do. The accounting and balancing of the books took a good two weeks to teach besides the other nursing duties. So I had asked my supervisor in January to get me someone from a nursing pool. He did not and I was becoming more and more stressed about that. My husband said, "Don't worry about it. That is their problem."

When my body crashed, the company managed to get one of the part-time nurses to come back and work full-time. She was not interested in working for my vacation. She was always too busy. So, yes, the company survived without me. Actually, I was happy she did because I knew she could do the job and I no longer had to be concerned about the clients or the job. This took a lot of pressure off of me and I could concentrate on my illness. Again my husband was right. Maybe I have been taken advantage of all these years when I worked with no days off.

Now the anger I had suppressed for so long started flowing out of me. I finally admitted it to my friend and to my sister. I told my friend that I was so angry and I did not know what to do about it. I felt this little voice inside saying, "forgive, forgive." One day my sister came over to visit. I was so irritable. I tried to just be quiet and I told her I have so much anger that I felt as though I would explode. I explained to her that it had nothing to do with her. I told her that I know I have to work on forgiveness and until I do, this anger would not be resolved.

I decided I needed to take a look at my belief system. How could I possibly be angry with the people at work when I readily accepted the responsibility? Why did I put others before myself? Just what was my belief system?

My belief was to put everyone before myself. I had to own that I did not treat my body very well. I did not do this on purpose. I believed to go the one step further even if it took my last breath was to serve others. Actually, my husband and I were sitting at the kitchen table and I asked him, "Just what do you mean when you say I do not care about myself?"

He replied, "You allow others to take advantage of you. If someone needs something there you go. When you are sick, you will go to work anyway. You stress about taking time off work because you say there is no one to cover for you and that is the company's responsibility, not yours."

Oh, I finally get it. Then I tell him that I am writing this particular chapter on what I believe and I know I am going to be shown something I never knew or something that I am not consciously aware of.

Suddenly I had a vision of myself as young child two and a half years old, standing on the back porch, watching my mom and dad come home from the hospital with my new baby brother. I was the eighth of ten children and when I was born there were five years between my older twin brothers and me, so as you can probably guess, I got a lot of attention.

Anyway, as the vision begins to unfold, I start crying and shaking. My husband does not have a clue, so I try to describe what I am seeing. I see myself standing on the back porch at two and a half years old. My mom and dad had just entered the driveway. My younger brother had just been born. I am actually in the present feeling those terrible feelings I had for my new baby brother. I did not want my brother to take my place. I scolded myself real well because I knew this was wrong to have these feelings and that I was being "selfish". Right then and there I said to God, "Please help me not to be "selfish" and I believed that those feelings were terrible, wrong and inexcusable.

I got upset with my dad when he made my twin brothers get off of my tricycle. I did not want to be a part of that. I wanted to share. I knew they had "used" bicycles and I had a new one; therefore, this was not fair. I would have rather they have new bikes than I. Again, I did not want to be "selfish".

I was very aware of my environment. I found myself helping and trying to keep peace. I remember when my sister was told she would get a spanking if she did not do the dishes; instead, she went over to her friend's house. I was about five years old. I got a chair and pulled it up to the sink. I thought I could get them done before my dad got home. As I tried to get the dishes done it seemed as though the stack got higher and higher. Needless to say, my sister and Dad had a very bad argument. I was sure that if I had got the dishes done everything would have been fine.

Another time I asked my mom, "Why do you have a headache when we have to go get groceries?" She told me that she had too much to do. I again asked, "What do you mean?" She said, "It is because there is so much to do. I have to get myself and your brothers ready before we can go." So I decided to give baths to my younger brothers and get them dressed.

As silly as this might seem, I prayed not to be selfish and at that time I decided I would help rather than be a burden to anyone. The day I was experiencing those terrible feelings about my brother, I made a vow not to bother God with my problems. I felt He had too many people to take care of and if I could help people rather than ask for help, His load would be lighter also. Thus my identity was established to be a caretaker.

I learned to discipline myself. I recall my mother said that I had "potty trained" myself. I would not allow myself to watch television if my homework was not done or I hadn't taken my bath. It was important that my clothes be ready for school the next day. My mom did not know this because she would say, "Your favorite show is on." I would tell her I would be there later. I found out that if I was tired at school, I needed to go to bed earlier. Isn't that ironic? I was aware of the sleep my body needed in order to be alert for school; but when it came to taking care of others I lost that sense of discipline.

In fact, when I became a nurse's assistant before I became a nurse; I could not believe people actually got paid for helping others. I loved it. It was most certainly my spiritual mission.

I correlated that with raising my children in a religious atmosphere. It was a priority to me that they go to a parochial school. My ex-husband said to me, "Just look at that money you are spending on schooling when these children could have more things and you could have decent furniture." I explained to him that I was more concerned about a God given spirit than of anything in this world.

Sometimes I worked two jobs to achieve what I wanted for my children. I had this great sense of responsibility to my children and my job. I was the one who believed that if I did not go to work these clients would not be medicated. All of these beliefs were only mine. I was the one who did not set limits. I was the one who did not know about healthy boundaries. Yet my intent was good. I truly loved to help.

You see I established this belief system as a young child. I scolded that child for the terrible feelings I had for my new baby brother. I can, as an adult, put labels on those feelings such as envy, fear of abandonment and fear of not being loved anymore. I even shamed that child for those terrible feelings. I knew I never wanted to be "selfish" again. The one thing I could do now was to tell God I would help Him. I will help take care of other people as I said earlier to lighten His load. As that little girl, I made a vow not to put myself first and not to ask for help. I could do it myself. So all of my life I have dedicated myself to others and I have always felt so good about it. I never felt I was a martyr and I never felt I did it to be accepted by people. A family member told me that I only helped people to be accepted and that I begrudged it later. This was not true for me.

I remember a psychologist asking me why I felt so unworthy. He said it was not a matter of low self-esteem but that of shame. Now when I look back I realize whom I had to forgive. It was me. I had to forgive myself for condemning myself for those "terrible" feelings I experienced toward my little brother. I made "a conscious decision about my feelings toward my brother that was not acceptable or excusable and therefore I was unworthy to live" which is, in a nutshell, the definition of shame.

Upon this realization I cried and cried and cried because I love that little girl. I love her innocence and her consciousness. Perhaps I thought I had lost my identity with this illness, but now with this realization about forgiveness, I know who I am and have been all my life. I am proud to be a servant to the people. I am proud of my values as a child. I now know there is nothing in this world to forgive. People talk and live from their belief system.

Now as I examine the incident with my job and hear the words that were said about me, I may be hurt but I cannot be angry any more with these people who do not know who I am. Most of all, spiritually I have realized that there is nothing to forgive. I suggest from my own insight that forgiveness is never about someone else. It is about you. It is your belief system.

The little voice inside saying "forgiveness, forgiveness" was there for me to forgive myself, to reconnect with my true identity and also to realize no matter what happens to me I will never ever lose my identity for I know who I am.

Living With Limitations

"The unexamined life is not worth living."
Socrates

Forgiveness was just one step in the process of self-realization. I recognize that this chronic illness is a gift. I decided to see the glass half full rather than half empty. I needed to learn how to live my life with quality and creativity.

The past year I had lived with attending doctor appointments and therapy. I had to spend the rest of the day resting with a heating pad and medication. The other days I occupied myself with crocheting, cross-stitching, jigsaw puzzles and cryptograms. Sometimes I would listen to music or read a good book.

Television was not a priority, but I did enjoy a good wholesome old fashioned movie. I preferred drama or mysteries. All of these activities were fun, yet lacking socialization. My family and friends called and we would talk and it was great. They were and are my support system. I am so grateful to have family and friends that care what is going on in my world even though I was not active in their world.

I decide it is time I try to go on a trip with my husband. We have a trailer on a camp ground up north and he loves to fish. He is very aware of my limitations. I put the seat back when my abdomen would start to distend. We stopped frequently. Time was of no essence. He was retired and has a bad back, which reinforced the need to stop and get out and stretch.

The trip turned out to be wonderful. When we first got there, I was exhausted and my abdomen was hurting. I knew how to cope with this as I learned at home from any activity. There were times I could not go in the boat and the times I did were short. I had brought my crocheting, books, and movies. I knew I could entertain myself. This was great. I discovered how to travel and what to expect and how to deal with my illness. I was certainly amazed that I did not have to stay home all of the time.

The holidays were coming. I usually fixed one dinner either for Christmas or Thanksgiving. This year I volunteered for one of the dinners as usual. My oldest daughter would fix the other dinner. My younger daughter and sister offered to come over and help me. I told them it was not necessary and told them my plan. I thought if I could prepare some of the food the day before I would not have so much to do in one day. I was sure that would work. Even though I worked on the dinner the day before I was so exhausted I really did not enjoy the visiting. In fact, I will not be cooking at all this year unless it is one simple dish.

I realized I could work in my flower garden thirty minutes comfortably and sixty minutes at the max. Sixty minutes required the whole scenario, the sofa, the heating pad, medication and plan on staying there the rest of the day and possibly the next day.

I have two sisters and a brother who bowl in a senior league. It is not a regular sanctioned league. You did not compete to win, you just bowled. My sisters invited me to have lunch with them after they bowled. They always signed up for the lunch that was served at the bowling alley. Here I go and I am excited to see them bowl and certainly looking forward to visiting. I enjoyed it more than I thought. I got so excited watching them bowl it was as if I was bowling too. I was welcomed to do this every Tuesday. I knew that to go every Tuesday that I would not exert myself on Monday. This prompted me to search for other social activities I could attend.

I found out there was a book club every other Thursday of the month. The book club only lasted an hour. The book was about the very subject I loved the most, living a better life spiritually. There were ten people in the group and it was intriguing listening to each person's interpretation of the book. This opened my mind to become the observer and listener. Most of all, I learned that each moment is an opportunity to be grateful for my life and that I am a co-creator of the moment. My life could be as fulfilling as I wanted it to be.

My brother and his girlfriend invited my husband and me to an arthritis water therapy class. We went to one of the classes. My husband was not interested. I was, so I joined. I go to this water therapy three times a week for twenty minutes. The exercise not only helped my body; it also increased the endorphins and I could tell right away that my mental status was more positive. This does not mean that my muscles did not spasm, they did. I knew what to do to help myself with the pain. I acknowledge that I will have pain and spasms with different activities. That is why the illness is chronic, but it is also manageable.

I decided take a short trip with a friend of mine to visit a church. She was worried about my well being. I assured her I could manage the pain. By the time we got to the hotel, my abdomen was much distended. I had taken pain medication before we got there and that helped a lot. The swelling of the abdomen was inevitable. I was exhausted and uncomfortable. I knew I had to lie down for a while.

The next morning I was refreshed. We went to hear a pastor speak about the "no complaint" purple bracelet. I had seen this man on the Oprah show not long ago. The theory behind his bracelet was that you wear it on one wrist. If you complain, you have to put it on the other wrist. The goal is to keep the bracelet on one wrist for twenty-one days. The pastor said he had heard it takes twenty-one days to develop a habit; therefore, wearing the bracelet for twenty-one days would change a person's thought process. It most certainly is a good idea. Can you imagine our world with no complaints? He gives the bracelets away. He has already given bracelets to eighty different countries. His web site is http://www.nocomplaintbracelet.org.

What an inspiration for me spiritually, especially at this time of my life. It helped me become more aware of all of the things I had to be grateful. The drive home was another realization.

My friend asked me a question and I answered, "That is fear. What are you afraid of?" Tingles ran up my spine to the top of my head. I realized the answer did not come from an intellectual insight. It came from the voice within. I knew right away that this question about fear pertained to me as much as it did her. She said, "I would have never thought of that." I said, "I know this is true, because when I experience tingles I know that I did not say it. This was given to me before I could think about the answer." What a question! I thought to myself, why and what am I afraid of? I had learned in one of my spiritual classes and also in a book I read that there are only two emotions; fear and love. That is when I began to see I had lived my entire life out of fear. I parented my children out of fear. I taught them to be afraid. I wondered what my fears were.

Embrace My Fears

"What you resists, persists."
Carl Jung

It was Friday, the weekend of Easter, when we returned home. Unknowingly, each of us had decided independently, to find a church in our area similar to the one we visited. My friend called me Saturday night and said, "I found a church in town similar to the one we visited. I decided I would go tomorrow."

I said, "You have? I was thinking about finding one myself."

"Do you want to go?" she asked.

"I would love to next week. This weekend Paul and I have plans."

As soon as we came home, I called my friend to find out about the church. She was very pleased with the church, so we agreed to meet the following Sunday to have coffee before church.

I enjoyed the church as much as she did. Right away I registered for some classes that were being taught. I enjoyed the classes and the people. Yet, the conversation I had with my friend about fear nagged at me night and day. I had to ask myself what were my fears?

Fear, as defined in Funk and Wagnall's Standard Dictionary, is '*The possibility that something dreaded or unwanted may occur. To be uneasy or apprehensive*' and the other definition is '*an agitated feeling aroused by an awareness of actual or threatening danger or trouble, etc.*'

I reminded myself that throughout my life I had been afraid. I realized when I was afraid it was because I was experiencing a change. I can recall being afraid when I entered the first grade, the first time I tried to ride a bike, and the first time I rode on a bus or flew in an airplane. The list could go on and on. So what were my fears?

I had been apprehensive about my illness. I did not know what was wrong and it appeared that no one else did either. No one could answer the questions about my illness like whether it was chronic or acute.

In fact, I was treated like I was invisible by some medical professionals. I was not given respect as a person. Thus, the title of my book was created. I named my chapters of this book to begin with each letter in the word *invisible.*

I was beginning to have doubt about many aspects of my life. Fear thrives on doubt.

I was afraid of isolation. After all, my contact with people was at work. Most people I knew were working and even so, I could not sit up for more than thirty minutes.

What if I could never work again? How would I survive financially? I had a savings account; but I knew I could not live on that forever. How long would it be before I knew if I could go back to work?

I was afraid that my relationship with my husband would end. After all, I could not contribute financially and I could not do the household chores, yard work or errands.

Now, as I was physically unable to function as a nurse the questions were, what is my mission and who am I? I am a mother, wife, grandmother, sister, daughter, etc. yet, what was my mission? All of these fears were related to my illness. I could not address any of these fears until I completed my search for medical help.

Because of my illness, I was afraid my relationship with my husband would end. After all, he married a person who was independent. I contributed to the household financially and I was able to do the household duties and errands. Now, he did everything. He retired, two years prior to my illness, because he became disabled. He had to learn to live on a limited amount of money and limited amount of activity. Now I needed help. I saw myself as a burden. I became more apprehensive when he told me what the bills were. I was sure he perceived me as a burden.

When he spoke of money in any way I would become sarcastic. Finally after six months of torturing myself, I said, "I think it would be the best for both of us for me to move. I have thought about this for a while and I know I can get an apartment and live on my savings until I receive disability."

He said, "Why do you want to move?"

"Because," I answered, "I know that you think I am a burden."

"I do not think such a thing," he said. "Isn't that what being married is all about? Accepting the good as well as the bad?"

"Yes," I said, "but I know how afraid you are of not having enough money and I cannot contribute anymore."

He answered, "That is ridiculous." I knew he was right. He meant what he said and I knew it was the truth. That was another belief I had as a child. I discovered by helping I felt I was earning my way.

It took ten months and ten different doctors who gave me several diagnoses. Since my illnesses could not be cured, my condition was chronic. The symptoms were unpredictable and limited my physical capabilities. I learned how to live with my limitations and manage my pain for short periods of time.

Socially, I discovered I could go to water therapy for twenty minutes. I could join a book club. I only had to attend once a week and if I could not stay for the entire hour it was okay. If my symptoms were severe, I did not have to go to water therapy or to the book club. I could go to church or not depending on my symptoms. My fear of isolation was obliterated.

Financially, I applied for social security disability. I was rejected two times and I hired an attorney to request a hearing. I did not know when I would receive disability. I was eighty percent sure I would so I was less apprehensive.

Wow, I said to myself, what a realization! I identified my worth by what I contributed and I perceived he thought of me in the same way. This was why I was having the nightmares of being homeless and why I became apprehensive when he spoke of the bills. I felt he was pouring salt in a wound. The wound was my disability which I could not change.

Another fear was who am I? I am not a nurse or at least I cannot work as a nurse. Then I realized I could say I am a wife, mother, grandmother, great-grandmother, sister, daughter, etc. It finally dawned on me; I am a spirit experiencing life in a human body. I have nothing to fear. Fear is doubt and I choose to live in faith.

I do believe what my dad taught me, that is, when one door closes, another opens. He said, "Everything happens for a reason. We may not see in our life time why it happened and then, again, we may. Either way, know whatever happens was for the best."

Once I began to address each fear, I began to see more clearly. I saw the many facets of fear such as, doubt, insecurity, lack of self worth, confusion, anger, emotional pain, rigidity, tunnel vision, control, judgment and the need to be right. I know these are only a few examples. I am sure there are many more.

It is ironic how, as a nurse, I recognized the patients who were labeled "difficult", "impatient", "grumpy" were good people who were afraid. I loved to take care of them. Not because as some nurses would say, "Give that patient to Becky. She has the patience of Job." It was because I knew what they needed. It was my job to find out what they were afraid of and to earn their trust. Yet, I did not recognize fear in myself and in other people around me. Fear is not bad. It is a road sign directing one to look within. I am so grateful for these journeys. As I journeyed on the outside to seek help for my body, I simultaneously took a journey within and both were equally educational and very valuable. I started with this quote; so, I will end with it as well:

> *"What lies behind us and what lies before us are small matters compared to what lies within us."*
>
> Ralph Waldo Emerson

Epilogue

"Your vision will become clear only when you look into your heart. Who looks outside, dreams, who looks inside, awakens."
Carl Jung

I recall a story my friend told me about "getting off of the wheel", and I have a good laugh. I can see the little hamster going around and around and around. It was a perfect description of my life before my illness. I did not know how to slow down, get off of the wheel and rest; therefore, my body made the decision for me.

The quote by Carl Jung is so true. I have been given the opportunity to look within. I have become an observer. I do see clearer, especially when it pertains to what I say or how I react.

I am learning to live in the moment. I do not succeed one hundred percent but I am aware when I am not. Living in the moment there is a "peace that surpasses all understanding."

When I am tired, frustrated or have negative thoughts, I am not living in that moment. I have pushed beyond my physical limits and have to ask myself what is the fear?

The majority of the time I love my life. In fact, I have a better relationship with my adult children. As my son said to me, "Mom, I just want you to listen. I don't want you to fix it." I have become a better listener than I have ever been. I can discern between drama, fear and insecurity. One day my daughter Laurinda said, "Mom, I bet you get tired of hearing about my problems." I can truthfully say, as my mother said to me when I asked her the same question, "I want to know what is going on in your life. You may talk about a problem and I do not solve it. You have the answer as you talk about it." That is truly a giant step for me. I was the type of mother that wanted to "fix it". Again, my illness taught me that I could not fix anything or control anyone.

I have learned what is important and what is not. Perceptions I have had over the past years of my life were exactly that, perceptions. They are not truths. Truth does not perceive, judge, criticize and truth does not change. I know that acceptance of myself precedes acceptance of others. By accepting myself and others there is nothing to forgive.

Adversity or challenges promote opportunities to live a better life or a better way of thinking. The greatest realization for me is that I had always identified myself by what I could do. Now, it is as if this big burden of doing is gone and I am allowed to just be. I do not allow what other people say or think to upset my world.

In fact, I had a conversation with my daughter, Angela and she was concerned about what someone had said. She said, "Mom, I was in a great mood and had my day planned. When I heard this, I became so upset."

I said, "Do not let anyone or circumstance take away your peace. Do not allow the world to dictate to you how you should react in the moment. Do not give your power away."

"Thanks mom, I feel better already. That is the best advice you ever gave me. I feel like I have a secret."

Yes, I thought to myself. We all have a secret and that is each person is a unique individual. It is in knowing that I am Spirit experiencing living as a human being. My life will be as fulfilling as I want it to be. My life will be forever changing, creating and growing.

Perhaps I do know who I am. I am grateful for my illness, to the medical professionals and others who did not believe me. This was the perfect opportunity for me to journey within and find the greatest gift of all; I have awakened and am very much aware of who I am.

Information about Irritable Bowel Syndrome, Pelvic Floor Dysfunction and Interstitial Cystitis

It has been two years since I was diagnosed with interstitial cystitis, irritable bowel syndrome and pelvic floor dysfunction. Although I was diagnosed over a ten month period and each of the illnesses were diagnosed separately, these conditions are more commonly seen together. Other diseases related to these are Fibromyalgia, chronic fatigue syndrome, and Crohn's disease as well as Lupus just to name a few.

If I would have been told by a physician exactly that, I would not have lived ten months wondering how I was going to survive, is there a cure and what can I tell my employer.

When I would ask these questions, I was judged that I was hinting for the physician to say I was disabled and therefore, I was not educated and treated holistically. I had a psychological exam that was required by social security. I heard the results of that when the judge read what the psychologist stated. It was said that I felt I must be the only person in the world to have these problems. Yes, I did think that because I was not told these conditions are commonly seen together and that they were chronic conditions which were treatable but not curable.

So, yes I had what the book, *A Headache in the Pelvis, by Dr David Wise and Dr. Rodney Anderson,* describes as "catastrophic thinking" meaning thinking pessimistically about my condition. It also meant thinking that I may never get well and living in fear because questions I asked needed answering. Living in fear when the physician tells you, "I have no idea why you are having pain. My other patients do not." This causes more tension and anxiety which causes more pain. I do believe what the book states about doctors needing to talk and relate with each other in the different specialties of medicine. I also believe even if they do not communicate, they need to listen to what the patient states the other physician discovered. I am sharing this with you because in the crisis of severe pain, I could not walk, or sit up at all. I could not do research because I could not concentrate. I remained in confusion due to the lack of communication and education. I am going to give you the information about Interstitial Cystitis, Pelvic Floor Dysfunction and Irritable Bowel Syndrome as described by Mayo clinic's website, bio-medical.com and by the Interstitial Cystitis Association.

Irritable Bowel Syndrome

Irritable bowel syndrome is one of the most common disorders that doctors diagnose.

It is not talked about because some people are embarrassed by the signs and symptoms.

As many as one in five people in the United States have this disorder. It does not increase your risk of colon cancer and can be managed by diet, lifestyle and de-stressing techniques.

Signs and symptoms are:

- Abdominal pain
- A bloated feeling
- Gas
- Diarrhea or constipation Sometimes alternating between the constipation and diarrhea
- Mucus in the stool

Many people may have only mild signs and symptoms. Some people have such severe signs and symptoms that do not respond well to medical treatment and sometimes because it is complicated with other diseases. Most of the time it is noted to be a chronic condition.

Normally the muscles of the intestines contract and relax in a coordinated rhythm. In irritable bowel syndrome the muscles' contractions may force food too quickly through the intestine and the opposite can occur which is diarrhea.

Some researchers believe it is caused by changes in the nerves that control the muscle sensation or contractions in the bowel. People with irritable bowel may have a heightened sensitivity to stretching of the bowel with gas leading to pain and bloating. Others believe it is due to the central nervous system.

Some triggers may be stress, food or lactose intolerance.

Because there are usually no physical signs to definitively diagnose irritable syndrome, diagnosis is often a process of elimination.

Research has developed diagnostic criteria, of which the most important are abdominal pain and discomfort lasting at least twelve weeks. Others are:

- A change in the frequency or consistency of your stool.
- Straining, urgency or a feeling that you cannot empty your bowels completely.
- Mucus in your stool
- Bloating or abdominal distension.

Other red flags are:

- New onset after age 50
- Weight loss
- Fever
- Recurrent vomiting

If the red flags are present the doctor may elect to do additional testing.

Some additional tests could be flexible sigmoidoscopy (looking at the lower part of the colon with a flexible lighted tube.)

Other tests include: Colonoscopy and or abdominal x-rays of the internal organs which help the doctor to rule out other conditions of your symptoms.

There are Lactose intolerance tests which may be needed. Lactase is an enzyme you need to digest the sugar found in dairy products. Lacking this enzyme you may have similar symptoms of irritable bowel such as abdominal pain, diarrhea and gas.

Blood tests to see if you are allergic to wheat protein also may cause the symptoms of irritable bowel.

In my case I did have the CT (x-ray) of the abdomen and a colonoscopy and a motility tests.

My bowel has not moved on its own for several years. The doctor had me wait five days after trying fiber and other medications which only caused more bloating and pain. I also have other diseases that complicate this diagnosis. The CT was normal as well as the colonoscopy. The motility test proved that my colon moved very slowly which, in turn, encouraged the constipation. I have to use laxatives every other day at this time.

There are many suggested ways one can help this condition by paying attention to what you eat that causes the pain or bloating of the abdomen. Drink plenty of fluids. Exercise, biofeedback, deep breathing, experiment with fiber and eating at regular times are some of the suggested ways to help reduce symptoms.

Pelvic Floor Dysfunction

I have found information from Dr. Moldwin who is an Assistant Professor of Urology at the Albert Einstein College of Medicine and is Director of the Interstitial Cystitis Center at Long Island Jewish Medical Center in New Hyde Park, NY. He defines pelvic floor dysfunction as he first gives the definition of the pelvic floor muscles.

He states that the pelvic floor muscles support the organs of the body such as the bladder, rectum and uterus. The muscles of the pelvic floor are very broad based and act as a hammock for the organs. He states that the function of the muscles is to relax and contract to allow body functions such as urinating and having a bowl movement. They also contract when a person is walking around so one does not urinate at the same time. The physiologies of these muscles are so complex and he is not aware of any study that has examined this complexity of physiology at this time.

Pelvic floor dysfunction is uncoordinated behavior of the pelvic floor muscles. There is absolutely no relation to Parkinson's or multiple sclerosis. It is non-neurogenic. He states that when a person urinates, the muscle of the bladder contracts and forces out the urine and at the same time the other muscles of the pelvic floor have to relax. With pelvic floor dysfunction, the bladder opens up and yet, the urine does not come out because of the muscle spasms of other muscles.

He also compares pelvic floor dysfunction with interstitial cystitis as well as constipation due to the uncoordinated muscle contractions of the pelvic floor. They tend to have the same symptoms due to the pelvic pain, frequency and urgency to empty the bladder. Due to the muscle spasms of the rectum a person tends to become constipated.

Pelvic floor dysfunction is diagnosed by a physical exam. The pelvic floor muscles are examined by pushing the muscles at a seven o'clock and five o'clock positions. In pelvic floor dysfunction the patient grimaces or cries out in pain.

This was done to me by the physical therapist which validated my pain. The therapist is the one who explained that my muscles should feel soft and supple. Mine she said were "tight as guitar strings with knots in them." The pain I felt was very severe and I wanted to scream yet, I was so thankful that someone had found my pain. She was the one also that measured the relaxations of my pelvic muscles of which were very abnormal. In the resting state with my legs elevated I was comfortable; yet when I stood up and walked I had severe pain in my pelvis, lower back and thighs and buttocks.

Back to Dr. Moldwin's article, in which he states that he is very aggressive in treating constipation because constipation with the pelvic floor dysfunction stops the bladder from functioning.

(This does happen to me on a regular basis. I have to do deep breathing exercises to relax so that the bladder can empty. He also suggests warm baths on a regular basis which I learned helped my pelvic muscles to relax).

The other form of treatment is muscle relaxants. I take these at bedtime. He suggests biofeedback which I found to be very helpful along with myofascial/trigger point release. Myofascial trigger release is when the therapist has direct physical contact with the physical sites of pain and constriction. The objective is to stretch the muscles so that they can receive the proper oxygenation and nutrition and relief of the pain. This absolutely worked for me. I walked bent over in pain until I had this therapy. I could stand up straight and the pain was relieved for short intervals. Yet, I learned from the biofeedback to relax the muscles on my own, especially when I was aware of the tension. I do not recognize the tension one hundred per cent of the time until I am in pain. I have to learn to listen to my body.

Dr Moldwin states there is no known cause although this condition of keeping the pelvic floor muscles tight may have been started in childhood. It also could be caused by pushing and straining. The bladder is a muscle and by pushing and straining the rectal and abdominal muscles increase in pressure. That pressure is directed to the bladder and interferes with the bladder's natural state of contraction to urinate.

It is not known which disease came first, interstitial cystitis or pelvic floor dysfunction.

Due to pelvic floor dysfunction, I cannot walk or stand or sit for over an hour without pelvic pain and bloating of the abdomen. This disease cannot be cured but it can be managed with relaxation methods, muscle relaxants and by controlling my constipation with diet and medications. I do know my limitations and when I exceed those boundaries it takes longer to recuperate.

Interstitial Cystitis

Interstitial Cystitis, as defined by the Interstitial Cystitis Association is a chronic inflammatory condition of the bladder. It is not caused by bacteria and does not respond to antibiotics.

You may think you have a urinary tract infection because of the frequency, or urgency to urinate. Wherever you go the first thing you do is locate the nearest toilet. It is difficult to get a good night's sleep due to the pressure or pain in the bladder that awakens you.

Interstitial cystitis is a chronic condition that affects an estimated one million Americans. It does affect children and men but affects women the most. It can have a long lasting adverse reaction on a person's quality of life.

The severity of the symptoms can fluctuate and some people can experience periods of remissions. One may have all or some of the following symptoms:

- A persistent need to urinate, urinating as much as sixty times a day.

- Urgency is the need to urinate but cannot due to the spasms of the bladder, pressure and pain.
- Pain can be located in the lower abdomen. Pain can also be felt in the vaginal area and the urethra.
- The lining of the bladder wall is inflamed and is said by some theories that there may be a defect in the lining of the bladder. A leak in the lining may allow toxic substances in urine to irritate the bladder wall.

Other theories about what causes this condition include heredity, infectious or allergic condition but none has been proved.

The treatment available at this time is Elmiron. It is prescribed by the physician and taken orally as directed. It is believed to work by repairing a thin or damaged inner lining of the bladder. The other treatment available is bladder instillations of medication directly inserted into the bladder. This is a combination of medications that reduce the inflammation. These treatments have not been proven to help all people. There are no statistics about the success of these treatments.

I received both treatments and I cannot honestly say they worked at the time because of complications with pain in the pelvic floor muscles as well as the discomfort of abdominal distention. I do know that I had urgency, frequency and voided up to an average of fifteen times a day. The smallest amount was thirty ml. and the most as two hundred and fifty ml. The bladder can hold up to one thousand ml.

The other forms of treatment are relaxation techniques, elimination of acidic foods or drinks.

I hope that I have given enough information about these diseases that one can realize how symptoms of one can mimic another. I realized now how interrelated these organs and muscles are and it is more common than not to have two or three of these conditions.

Medical Terminology

Acute illness

An illness that has a sudden onset with severe symptoms and short course. The illness is usually diagnosed right away and usually has a cure.

Chronic Illness

An illness that persists for a long time. Symptoms may come and go unlikely to stay in remission. This illness has little if any progress over a long period of time. It is usually difficult to diagnose and may be treatable but not cured.

Adhesion

Union of two surfaces that are ordinarily separate; also any fibrous band that connects them. Surgery within the abdomen sometimes results in adhesions from scar tissue. As an organ heals, fibrous scar tissue forms around the incision. This scar tissue may cling to the adjoining organs causing them to kink. Adhesions are usually painless and cause no difficulties; although occasionally they produce malfunction or distortion of an organ.

Colon

Refers to the lower part of the intestines also known as the large intestine. It connects from the cecum (first bulging pouch of the large intestine) and ascends to the edge of the liver where it bends and becomes the transverse colon. This section lies across the abdominal cavity from right to left, below the stomach and then bends downward to become the descending colon. The descending colon extends downward on the left side of the abdomen. At the brim of the pelvis the colon extends in an 'S' shaped curve down to the sacrum where it becomes the rectum. The curved portion of the colon is called the sigmoid colon.

Colonic inertia

Weak muscular activity of the colon leading to distention of the organ and constipation. (Lazy colon)

Cystocele

Herniation or bulging of the urinary bladder.

Enterocele

Herniation or bulging of the intestine.

Rectocele

Herniation or bulging of the rectum.

Constipation

A condition in which the waste matter in the bowels is too hard to pass easily, or in which bowel movements are so infrequent that discomfort or uncomfortable symptoms result. Many people also use the term to refer to incomplete evacuation or when they feel they should have more bowel movements. The frequency of bowel movement varies according to individual body make-up, type of intestine, eating habits, physical activity and custom.

Herniated disc

There is a rubbery cartilage in between each vertebrae of the spine to cushion and absorb shock and allow movement. Excessive strain can cause the cartilage to bulge. Sometimes the bulging presses on the nerve root of the spinal cord causing pain.

Irritable Bowel Syndrome

A common disorder of the intestines that leads to cramping, bloating and changes in bowel habits. Some people have constipation (difficulty or infrequent bowel movements) and some people have diarrhea (frequent loose stools, often with an urgent need to have a bowel movement); some people have both and yet, some have the cramping and painful urge to move the bowels and cannot.

Gastroenterologist

A physician specializing in the stomach and intestines.

Interstitial Cystitis

A chronic inflammatory condition of the urinary bladder of unknown cause or causes. There is no specific sign or marker of the disease, so the diagnosis is made by excluding symptoms of other diseases. Symptoms may include urinary urgency and frequency, difficulty urinating and pain in the bladder and/or urethra that is temporarily relieved by voiding and/or pelvic pain. In some patients pain may radiate into the genitals, rectal and thigh areas. Urine cultures are negative (No urinary tract or bladder infection). If bladder is viewed with a scope ninety percent of patients will have ulcers, inflammation and some bleeding on the bladder wall.

Bladder Instillations

A combination of medication introduced into the bladder to help the pain and to promote healing of the bladder wall.

Pelvis

The lower portion of the trunk of the body, forming a basin bounded anteriorly and laterally by the hip bones and posteriorly by the sacrum and coccyx. The pelvis is subjected to more stress than any other body structure. The upper part of the pelvic girdle, which is somewhat flared, supports the weight of internal organs of the upper part of the body.

Pelvic Floor Dysfunction

The pelvis floor is the group of muscles that form a kind of sling or hammock that supports the pelvic organs, including the bladder, uterus or prostate, and rectum and surrounds the urethra, vagina (women) and the rectum. Those muscles have to be relaxed to urinate or have a bowel movement. With pelvic floor dysfunction, the muscles are tight or in spasm because of what is called the 'guarding reflex'. They have been tense because they are constantly fighting the urge to urinate or from the constant pain.

Physical Therapy

The treatment of bodily ailments by various physical or nonmedicinal methods. This usually includes the use of heat, water, exercise, massage and electric current.

Physical Therapist

One who is skilled in the therapeutic arts in the treatment of such disorders as fractures, sprains, muscle tension and paralysis.

Myofacial Release is a type of massage focused on trigger points that develop in muscles due to chronic pain or overuse. Therapist must have training for this specialty area

Urethra

A small tubular structure that allows urine to pass from the bladder out of the body. The female urethra is short in length compared to the male.

Ureters

The two fibro muscular tubes about nine inches long that transport the urine from the kidneys to the bladder.

Urinary bladder

It is a hollow sac that normally holds twelve to sixteen ounces of urine at a time (its functional capacity) although is capable of holding twenty five to thirty ounces (its true capacity). The bladder wall is composed of a thin mucous membrane lining, an epithelial lining, a layer of connective tissue and an outer muscular layer. It is controlled by both voluntary and involuntary muscles/nerves. Normally one needs to urinate every two to five hours.

Urogynecologist

A gynecologist who has a special interest in urinary problems of women.

Gynecologist

A physician who deals with diseases of the genital tract of women.

Urologist

A physician/surgeon who is trained to treat disorders of all organs and ducts involved in the production, release and elimination of urine i.e. Kidneys, ureters, bladder and urethra.

Disease Specific Associations and Web Sites

American Cancer Society

1599 Clifton Road NE

Atlanta, GA 30329

(800) 227-2345

www.cancer.org

American Chronic Pain Association

P.O. Box 850

Rocklin, Ca. 95677

(800) 533-3231

www.theapeu.org

Arthritis Foundation

1330 W. Peachtree St.

Atlanta, Ga. 30309

(800) 283-7800

www.arthritis.org

Fibromyalgia Network

P.O. Box 31750

Tucson, AZ. 85751

(800) 853-2929

www.fmnetnews.com

Interstitial Cystitis Association

110 North Washington St. Suite 340

Rockville, MO 20850

1-800-HELP ICA

www.ichelp.org

International Pelvic Pain Association

Suite 402

Brookward Medical Center Drive

Birmingham, AL 35209

(205) 397-9000

www.pelvicpain.org

National Institute of Health—NIH

The federal government agency that studies and funds research on diseases.

The National Institute of Diabetes and Digestive and Kidney Disease---NIDDK

This is a Section of NIH that funds bladder research including Interstitial Cystitis.

Web Site Resources

www.healinginmotion.com/womenshealth.htm

This site has information about pelvic pain and dysfunction.

www.beatprolapseandsiu.com

This site gives information about prolapses and stress incontinence.

www.pelvicpain.org/resources/2006

Presentations from the International Pelvic Pain Association

www.icnetwork.com/guestlectures/weiss

Dr. Weiss is answering questions about pelvic floor dysfunction.

www.mayohealth.com

General web site offers medical information about all illnesses.

www.bio-medical.com/news

Information about pelvic floor dysfunction.

www.improvingchroniccare.org

Foundation for improving chronic care.

www.health.nih.gov

National Institute of Health a very informative and disease specific therapies.

www.ichelp.org

Interstitial Cystitis Association.

Medical and Inspirational Books

A Delicate Balance Living Successfully With Chronic Illness, Susan Milstrey Wells Perseus Publications 2000.

This book is about a woman's personal journey after being diagnosed with Fibromyalgia, Sjogrens Syndrome and Interstitial Cystitis.

A Headache in the Pelvis, David Wise, PhD and Rodney Anderson M.D. National Center of Pelvic Pain 2003.

A new understanding and treatment for prostatitis and chronic pelvic pain syndrome.

For the Love of God, Edited by Benjamin Shield and Richard Carlson, New World Library, 19.

Actual teachings from the greatest spiritual leaders of the 20th century.

Life 10, John-Roger and Peter McWilliams, Publishers Press 1970.

Everything we wished we learned about in school but didn't.

Managing Pain Before It Manages You, Margaret A. Caudell, Guilford Press 2001.

Offers techniques you can apply immediately.

No More Sleepless Night, Peter Haurie, PhD and Shirley Linde PhD, Wiley 1996

Teaches you how to create your own sleep therapy.

The Power of Now, Eckhart Tolle, Publishers Group West 1999.

A Guide to Spiritual Enlightenment. Powerful doctrine teaching one to live in the moment.

The Seat of the Soul… Gary Zukav, Fireside 1990

Inspires one to realize the importance of life.

Teach Only Love, Gerald J. Jampolsky M.D. Beyond Words Publishing Co. 2000.

The twelve principles of attitudinal healing.

Tuesdays with Morrie, Mitch Album, Broadway Books 2002. Also in DVD.

A heart warming story of a college professor who is chronically ill. He shares his life lessons and wonderful attitude with a previous student.

Why People Don't Heal and How They Can, Carolyn Myss PhD, Harmony Books 1998.

She is a medical intuitive and teaches five myths people believe that if they would give them up, they would be on the road of healing.

You Don't Look Sick, Joy H. Selak and Steven S Overman M.D.MPH, Haworth Medical Press 2005.

Living well with a chronic illness. Joy's personal journey as she seeks for years to be diagnosed and treated. She and her doctor write the book together. She is diagnosed with Fatigue Syndrome, Interstitial Cystitis and Arthritis.

Author Biography

My name is Rebecca Kopp-DiPiazza. Kopp is my maiden name. I am the eighth child of ten children to be born into a Catholic family. I was the first child to be born in Rockford, Illinois.

My parents and siblings were born in Arkansas and moved to Rockford in 1950.

My father was raised Catholic and my mother was a Baptist who converted to Catholicism.

To know me, one must know my parents.

My parents were wonderful people. They had great work ethics. They were honest and believed children should be raised in a spiritual environment. My dad taught me my first prayers when I was a toddler. He was a humble and giving man. My brother told me that when they lived in Arkansas my father made wooden toys for the children of the town at Christmas. One day my brother asked my father what he was going to do with the piece of Mahogany wood. My father replied, "I am saving that for something special." Later on my brother tried to get into dad's workshop and it was locked. He found a way to open the lock He discovered a child's casket made of mahogany. Evidently there was a child who was dying in the small town where they lived. My dad never told me this story nor would he tell anyone.

My dad was a carpenter, musician, raised bees, farmer and most of all a man of great ethics and values. Any time I had questions his answers would be related to God or the Bible.

Once I asked him, "Dad why do we give the first of our crops to other people?" He replied without hesitation, "In the Bible it says that when one gives the first of their harvest away one will always have plenty. Now, haven't we always had plenty?"

I certainly could not argue with him. Dad went to church on Sundays and he said, "Anyone who wants to go to church must be up at 5a.m. (we lived on the farm and it took an hour to get to church.) My younger brother and I would be the ones to go.

I loved to be with my dad wherever he was. If he was working in the garden, tending the bees or working in his workshop, I would be there. When he went to jam sessions the entire family would go and we would dance. I loved to ask him what he was thinking.

One day he was standing on the front porch and I asked, "Dad what are you thinking about?" He replied, "I am praying for rain for the crops." I stood there with my head bowed and prayed also.

I was eight years old and for the first time I realized not all prayers were answered as expected.

Within the next month, dad and my twin brothers were putting in an irrigation system. Dad told me that everything works out for the best and followed that with, "When one door closes, another will open as long as you are doing the best you can."

My mother was raised Baptist. It was because of her diversity that she opened the door for me to explore other faiths. I attended the Catholic school for first grade and half of the second grade. I was told that I should not play with Protestants. I hurried home to ask mom, "Who are Protestants and why did the school tell me that I was not allowed to play with them?" She explained who Protestants were and that it was okay for me to play with my Protestant friends. I loved to go to the Pentacostal church across the street because they sang songs and I loved to sing. I also went to revivals that my friends had at their churches. I really believed I could not be saved enough.

One day my mom told me a story about judging people. She said, "I looked out the window and saw some children pulling a grown man in a wagon. I wondered why this man was so lazy that he had children pulling him in a wagon. As the wagon got closer I could see that the man did not have any feet. I made a promise to myself and that is from that day forward I would not judge anyone." She also added, "No one should judge another until he walks a mile in the other person's shoes." Mom cared about other people. It was not unusual for her to sit at the bedside of someone who was sick in the neighborhood. She also would say, "Just what do you think the neighbors would say?" And the other comment was, "We will have to wait until your dad comes home."

I wondered why she could not make the decision herself. I had a lot of questions as a child and was perceptive of disobeying before I could speak. We lived in the basement of the house my dad was building. I was a toddler and wanted to go upstairs. I would mumble to get mom's attention to tell her I was going. Most of the timed she caught me and brought me back down the stairs, yet, there were times I managed to make it. I was sure to tell her before I went.

Before I was school age, my Grandpa Chappell would call every morning. I would be the one to answer the phone so I could tell him everything and where each of my siblings were.

I would tell my younger brother where he could and could not go. In fact, after I became a teenager my younger brother told one of his friends, "If you can make it past Becky, the family will really like you."

When I was three years old and my brother was born was when I decided that mom and God had too many people to take care of therefore, I became a caretaker. This was a very natural place for me long before I became a nurse. At five years old I had a near death experience.

The family was at a local forest preserve and my dad was holding me in the water and he would let go and tell me to kick my feet and move my arms. I went down once, twice and the third time I was swirling through a dimly lit tunnel backwards. At the end of the tunnel was a very bright light and I saw on a huge screen (like a drive-in theater) my life pass before me.

I saw myself playing with my friends and then I saw myself stealing a piece of bubble gum at the local grocery store. I knew I must be dead and I said to God, "I didn't know you knew that." I laughed because I did not feel any rejection or judgment. Then I heard a voice telepathically say, "Are you ready to come?" Looking around I wanted to see where the origin of the light was coming. I could not see because the light was so bright, yet it did not hurt my eyes. I also looked for angels. I did not see any but I did hear the most beautiful tones of music that I have never heard before and even to this day. I suddenly saw my mom and dad and all of my brothers and sisters. I did not want to leave because I felt so much love from the light that encompassed me like a cocoon. I laughed again and said, "I am just a child. I have not lived yet." I felt my dad lift me out of the water and I ran to shore. I did not tell anyone until I was eleven years old. That is when I had heard that other children had the same experience. After the incident I did not believe in a punitive God.

The next year I entered the first grade at the Catholic school. When I opened my Catechism book I saw the rays of the sun shining through the trees and it reminded me of the God light I had seen. Academically school was easy. In fact I was promoted in the second grade to a higher second grade because the work was too easy. We moved to the farm in Arkansas in the middle of second grade. We did not finish the year of school. I was promoted to the third grade anyway. I attended the third through the seventh grade in Arkansas. My family moved back to Rockford Illinois in 1964. I attended junior high and completed high school in Rockford.

I was married in 1968 and our first daughter, Angela was born in 1970. We had our second daughter, Laurinda in 1972. That was the year my parents moved to California. We moved to California in 1974 and our son, Matthew was born in Bakersfield, California.

In 1975, I attended cosmetology school and graduated. I took my cosmetology test in Hollywood, Ca. My mom was my model. I passed and secured a job in a town near by. Within three months I had abdominal surgery. I had complications so I was in bed for the next six months.

After recuperating, I decided to apply for a job at the county hospital. I knew I did not have the artistic ability to be a cosmetologist. They offered to train me for a Certified Nurses' Attendant. I had no idea that I would have so much fear. I had told them that I could learn anything. Due to my shyness around strangers, my instructor had to literally take me by the hand and lead me into the patient's room to take the blood pressure. My fear was so bad that the only reason I stayed was because my dad had invested $20.00 in my stethoscope.

I knew I could not let him or my children down. I wanted to send my children to parochial school. There was no way I could quit now.

My first patient was dying and my instructor told me to come and get her when I recognized labored breathing. I managed to give him a bath and change the bed and then his breathing became so labored. I ran to my instructor and we went back to the room. I saw my instructor makes the sign of the cross right before he died. She explained to me that she had just baptized this man because she did not know if he had ever been baptized. I really liked my instructor. She was very compassionate and she taught me to always speak to the patients even if they were in a coma.

I loved my job. I wrote to my brother, "Imagine getting paid to help people, I feel as though I am stealing." The nurses encouraged me. They told me I would be a good nurse. I told them I could not afford to go to school. One of them gave me the name or an organization (CETA). She told me that they would pay for my education to become a nurse. I called the organization right away and make an appointment to go the office to see if I qualified. The man took my application and told me that there would be a test given in a little town thirty miles away and there were seventy people that would be taking the test. He also told me that it would be a waste of time for me to go because they were catering to the minority. I am low income how much more of a minority do I need to be. I went anyway. I tested high in the class of seventy. Twenty four were chosen. The twenty four had to take math, English and anatomy. Twelve top students would go into the L.V.N. (Licensed Vocational Nurse) and the last twelve would take classes to become medical assistants. I received the highest grade in the class. I could not have been more pleased.

I recalled saying in grade school that I did not want to be a nurse and I remembered what a friend in cosmetology school said to me. She said, "Becky you would make a wonderful nurse." I remembered laughing and telling her I could not stand the site of blood. I do not believe in coincidences. I knew I was guided by God to become a nurse and I knew it was my mission.

Again, that was another thing my dad told me, "If you work or try all that you can, God will do the rest and He sure did. Nursing school was not easy but because I had taken the cosmetology course I knew the names of all of the bones and because I was a nurses' attendant I had learned how to do sterile dressing changes, tube feedings and even tracheotomy care. I received the highest clinical award. One of my teachers told me why she gave me an A. She reminded of the time I asked her for help with a patient who would stop breathing when I turned him on his side. The man was dying from cancer and I went to my instructor three times for help. She would tell me that she would come but she never did. I stood outside of the patient's door and ask God to remove my fear and to use my body to bathe this man and change his bed. Before I knew it the job was completed and my instructor came in. I told her we did just fine. The instructor said that she was afraid to take care of the dying patient that is why she did not come. Actually her fear was the normal response from most nurses when a patient was dying.

There were many times I volunteered to take care of the dying. To me it was a very holy time to care for a person. One of my patients was talking to her dead husband. She told him how much she enjoyed the music he was playing. She was staring at the bathroom door as she spoke. I did not see anyone. She began saying over and over, "I have to be forgiven."

I asked, "Why do you need forgiveness?" She told me and I held her hand and said, "God has forgiven you. He loves you unconditionally." She became very peaceful and died within thirty minutes. One of my patients in coronary care unit stopped breathing and I immediately started CPR. The nurses and doctors rushed to the bedside and relieved me. I saw my patient's adult children open the double doors to the unit. I immediately ushered them back to the waiting room. Within forty five minutes the doctor came to the waiting room and told the family that their mother was stable and they could see her for a few minutes. After they left my patient told me she had left her body and saw me with her children in the waiting room. She thanked me for comforting them and that she knew she had to come back and prepare them for her death. Those two incidents were among many in my nursing career.

Taking care of people was an even exchange. It has been very rewarding and they have taught me so much about the human spirit.

I believed being a nurse was a great honor and I called for God's help throughout my career. I believe He used me to help others. I could not have done the job without Him.

I also believed my children were on loan to me from God and I needed to provide them with a spiritual foundation just as my parents did with me. I entered them into a parochial school; yet, I taught them at the same time with what my parents had taught me. My children helped me to care for my Dad when he became ill.

My dad knew that I would have a difficult time when he died. He was my mentor. I saw my parents every day especially when dad became ill. He explained his death to me with these words, "Becky, have you ever been afraid that I would not take care of you and your brothers and sisters? Were you afraid when we moved down south?"

I said, "Of course not, Dad." Then he stated, "That is the way it will be when I die. I will be going ahead of all of you to prepare a place for you and the rest of the family. We will be together again." Even though I believed him, I was not ready for him to die. Actually I do not believe anyone can prepare to lose a loved one. What he said did help and I think of his words often for I know he is not far away. My dad died in 1982.

I continued to work at Bakersfield Memorial Hospital until 1985 and moved back to the Midwest. I made a promise to my husband that we would move closer to his parents. In 1985 a Licensed Vocational Nurse could not buy a job. I happen to know someone who worked in a nursing home. She told me that I could get a job filling in for nurses when they went on vacation. Once I worked there I created a job by being the medication nurse for all three floors to relieve some of the work for the nurses in charge. The Director of Nurses agreed for a trial period of one month. Before the month was over a full time position was available. I became the charge nurse for the Alzheimer patients. I worked there for two years and then I worked for the Nursing pools until I secured a job in a doctor's office in 1989.

In the doctor's office I learned to assist the doctor with exams as well as minor surgeries. I also did billing and transcribing. I had so many jobs in the office that I was never bored. In 1993 he closed his practice. I went back to the nursing pools and back to college and obtained my degree as a registered nurse.

I found a job at a clinic downtown part-time and I found a full time job working for an Urologist. These jobs lasted until 1996 and that is when my part-time job became my full time job. I was working at the same clinic when I became ill in 2006.

By 2007 I was still struggling to accept my illness and my compromised life. I needed to share my story. In doing so, I received inspiration and healing. My hope is that this book will bring hope and inspiration to others.

I try to teach my children what my dad taught me. I tell them that when one door closes, another will open. I tell them that life is a journey of peaks and valleys. I tell them that we may see in our life time why something happens and then again we may not; yet everything happens for the best. I tell them that there are gifts in life's challenges. I tell them that it is not what happens to us in this life but it is how we react to the challenges. That is what living on this earth is all about. It is about hope, faith and doing the best we can. As we face the many challenges of life we learn compassion for others. In compassion we find love and in love we find peace.

Printed in the United States
204025BV00003B/364-429/P

9 780980 178081